Power BI Academy
Volume 2
Healthcare

Create and Learn

Roger F. Silva

Skill Level: **Beginner**

Estimated time to complete: **2 hours**

Copyright © 2022 by Roger F. Silva – Create and Learn

All rights reserved. No part of this publication may be reproduced, distributed, or transmitted in any form or by any means, including photocopying, recording, or other electronic or mechanical methods, without the prior written permission of the publisher, except in the case of brief quotations embodied in critical reviews and certain other non-commercial uses permitted by copyright law. For permission requests, write to the publisher, addressed "Attention: Permissions Coordinator," at the address below.

This book and any link available are for educational and information purpose only, and the author does not accept any responsibility for any liabilities resulting from the use of this information, files or software mentioned in this material.

Roger F. Silva

contact.createandlearn@gmail.com

createandlearn.net

linkedin.com/in/roger-f-silva

Power BI version: 64-bit (February 2021)

ISBN: 9781695706354

Contents

Introduction 1

Get Started 3

    1.   The Patient Overview Dataset 3
    2.   Business Intelligence and Power BI 3
    3.   Power BI Products 4
    4.   Business Intelligence for Healthcare 5
    5.   Install Power BI Desktop 6
    6.   Launch Power BI Desktop 14

Get Data 21

Model data 25

Creating Custom Calculations 33

Dashboard Page 43

Big Numbers 51

Patients by Area 71

Patients by Month 75

Patient Satisfaction 81

Patient Table 91

Patient by City 101

Waiting Time 107

Filters 115

Text and Objects 127

Bookmarks 133

Phone Layout **141**

Sharing **143**

Next Steps **153**

Final words **155**

Find more **Create and Learn** books
https://www.createandlearn.net/:

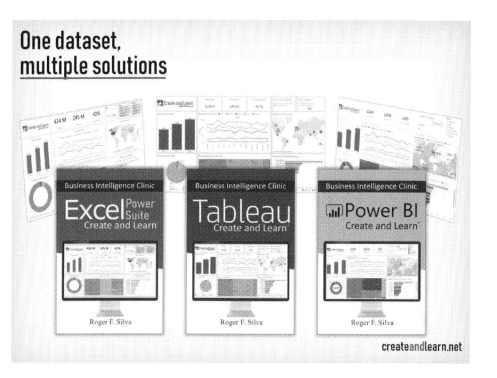

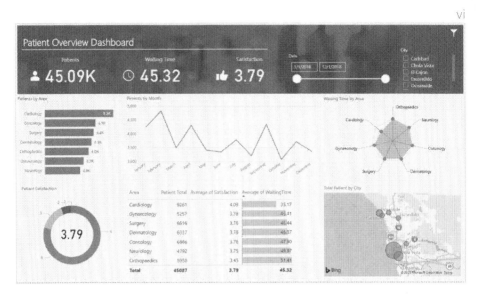

Dashboard to be created: **Patient Overview**

Introduction

Dear Reader,

Power BI Academy is a series of short books that help students and professionals improve their Power Business Intelligence (BI) knowledge by creating professional dashboards through quick step-by-step instructions.

Through this series, you will have the opportunity to work with datasets, metrics, and Key Performance Indicators (KPIs) from a wide range of industries, helping you become a valuable resource to any team and industry.

In this book, **Power BI Academy vol.2 – Healthcare**, which has over 200 images, you will learn to create a unique Dashboard for the Healthcare Industry.

You go through important topics of Microsoft Power BI Desktop, a Free BI tool from Microsoft. You will learn how to **install** Power BI Desktop, **get data** from Excel, **model** your Data, work with **visuals and reports**, create a **Patient Overview Dashboard**, and **share** your work.

We will not go into deep theories as to the purpose of this book, and all Create and Learn material is to make the most of your time and learn by doing.

You will follow step-by-step instructions to create a professional Healthcare Dashboard to help you rapidly increase your knowledge.

I also hope this book will help start your journey in the Business Intelligence world and provide the necessary tools to create professional reports and dashboards using Microsoft Power BI.

You can find more books and information on the website createandlearn.net/pbi

Thank you for creating and learning.

Roger F. Silva

contact.createandlearn@gmail.com
createandlearn.net
linkedin.com/in/roger-f-silva

Chapter 1

Get Started

1. The Patient Overview Dataset

The **Patient Overview** dataset is a friendly and easy-to-manage group of tables containing a fictional hospital's data.

These are the tables you will find:

Patient: Contains the overall details of each patient.

Satisfaction: Contains the score (ranging from 1 to 5) that each patient gave the hospital.

2. Business Intelligence and Power BI

Business Intelligence's primary goal is to help people and companies make better decisions, and according to Wikipedia, business intelligence is a set of methodologies, processes, architectures, and technologies that transform raw data into meaningful and useful information used to enable more effective strategic, tactical, and operational insights and decision-making.

Power BI is a Business Intelligence software that allows users to get data from multiple sources, transform the data, and create reports, dashboards, and many types of visualizations.

The user can share those reports with colleagues and customers across multiple platforms, such as Power BI service, SharePoint, websites, and more.

Until recently, Business Intelligence solutions were aimed at Enterprise-level BI with complex, costly products, and most of it was done by IT professionals.

Today, you can find a range of self-service BI solutions, and Power BI is one of them. These solutions allow analysts, managers, and various professionals to get data, model the data, create visualizations, and share them.

3. Power BI Products

According to Microsoft, Power BI is a suite of business analytics tools that deliver insights throughout your organization. It allows you to connect to hundreds of data sources, simplify data preparation, and drive ad hoc analysis. You can produce beautiful reports and publish them for your organization to access on the web and across mobile devices.

Power BI Desktop: <u>This program is the primary software used in this book</u>. Power BI Desktop is a free solution installed on the computer that allows users to connect the data, prepare and model the data, create reports, and run advanced analytics.

* The Power BI Desktop version used in this book is the 64-bit from September 2019.

Power BI Pro: It allows the user to access all the Power BI service content. The user will access an online portal, where it is possible to create dashboards, share with other Pro users, and publish on the web.

Power BI Premium: It provides dedicated resources to run Power BI for organizations or teams. It gives greater data volume, improved performance, and more widespread distribution.

Power BI Mobile: It offers apps for mobile devices. With mobile apps, users can connect and interact with both on-premises and cloud data.

Power BI Embedded: It integrates Power BI visuals into custom applications. Essentially, it enables companies to use all Power BI visuals and functions inside their applications as if they were native.

Power BI Report Server: It is the on-premises solution, and users can move to the cloud when they need it.

4. Business Intelligence for Healthcare

With the increasing number of data sources and the complexity of data generated within healthcare organizations, there is a growing need for advanced analytics to support the decision-making process.

Business Intelligence for healthcare is critical to managing the massive amounts of both structured and unstructured data that healthcare institutions deal with daily.

Additionally, BI can help organizations and administrators track KPIs that provide actionable insights regarding clinical, financial, and operational aspects.

The following are examples of trackable metrics to improve results for healthcare organizations:

Patient satisfaction

Patient stay

Overall and detailed costs

Readmission rates

Patient safety

Wait time

5. Install Power BI Desktop

To install Power BI Desktop in your computer, go to the Microsoft Power BI website. Currently, the address is **powerbi.com**, or you can search for "Power BI" inside the Microsoft main page, which is microsoft.com.

You will see multiple links to get the free version on the Power BI website, such as **Start Free**, **Sign up free**, and others.

1. Go to Products and select **Power BI Desktop** as the image below.

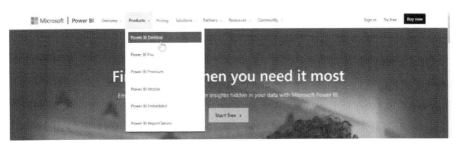

2. Then, click on **Download Free**.

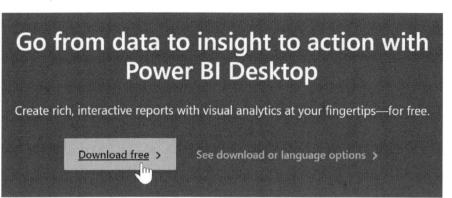

3. If the site redirects you to the Microsoft store, click **Install** to start the download and the install process.

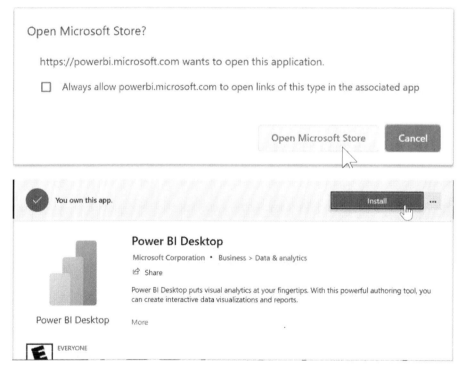

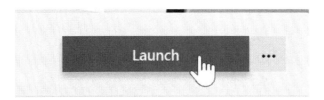

4. If you have installed Power BI, go to **Launch Power BI Desktop** chapter. If not, go to the next step.

5. If you want to download in any different language than English, click on **Advanced Download Options**, and select the language. If not, go to the next step.

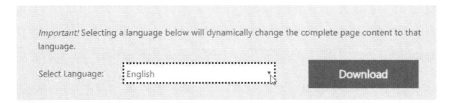

6. If the **Choose the download you want** message appears, select the windows version (usually is x64) and click on **Next**.

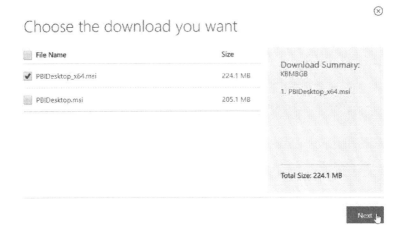

Get Started

7. After starting the install process, the setup screen will appear. Click on **next**.

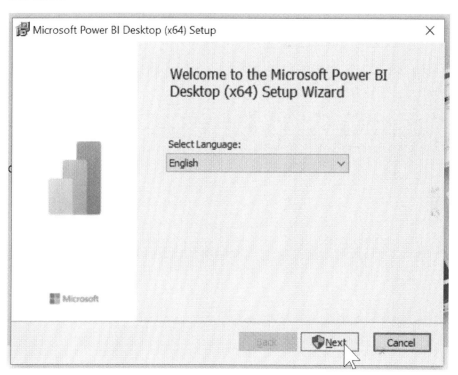

8. Read the license agreement, and if you agree, check the box "I accept the terms and license agreement" and click on **Next**. Also, you have the option to print.

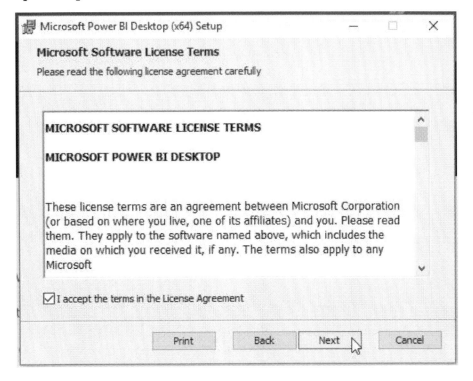

9. Click **Install**.

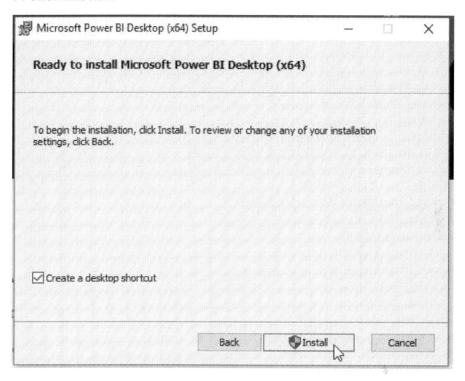

10. Check if you need to click **Yes** to allow Power BI to install and wait till the installation finishes.

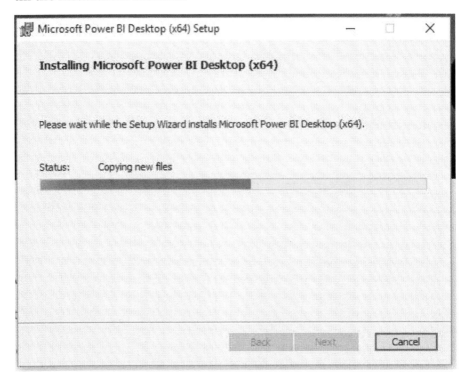

11. Once the installation is completed, leave the box "Launch Microsoft Power BI Desktop" checked and click **Finish**.

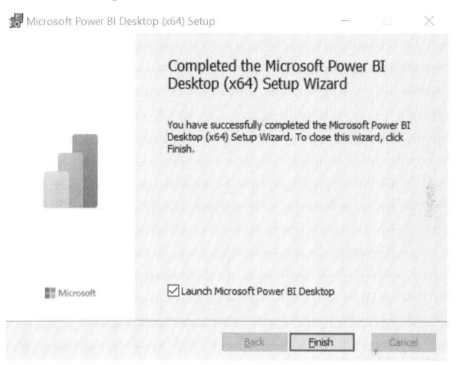

6. Launch Power BI Desktop

1. Once you launch Power BI, it will ask you to create a free account.

If you don't want to create an account now, click on **Already have a Power BI account** (bottom) and close the login window.

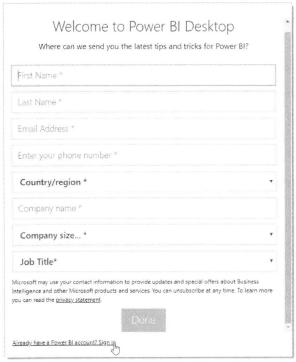

Get Started

2. Below you will find the start screen, and from here, you can start a new report using the **Get data**, access your recent/pinned reports, **sign in** to your powerbi.com account or **try it free**. Click on the right top and close this window.

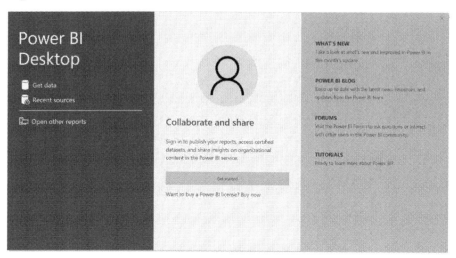

3. The image below shows the first view of Power BI, I will quickly introduce it to you, and as you build your reports, you will get used to most of its tools.

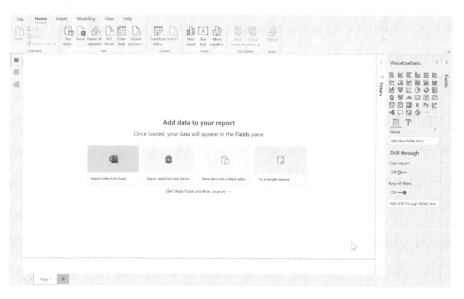

4. The **File** tab is the same that you find in most Microsoft products, where you can create, save, and export your file.

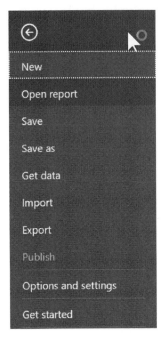

5. The **ribbon** displays common tasks related to visualizations and reports.

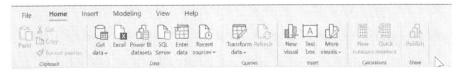

6. The Page tab along the bottom allows you to select, edit, or add a page.

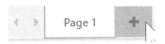

7. The **Report** view, or canvas, where visualizations are created/arranged, followed by **Data** view, where you will find your data, and **Model** (Relationships**)** view, where you can manage data relationships.

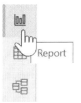

8. The **Visualizations** pane is the place where you can select visualizations, change colors or axes, drag fields, filters, and more. The **Fields** pane is the place that queries elements, and filters can be dragged to the Report view and Filters area. The **Filter** pane allows you to create faster filters to be used in a single page or multiple pages across the file.

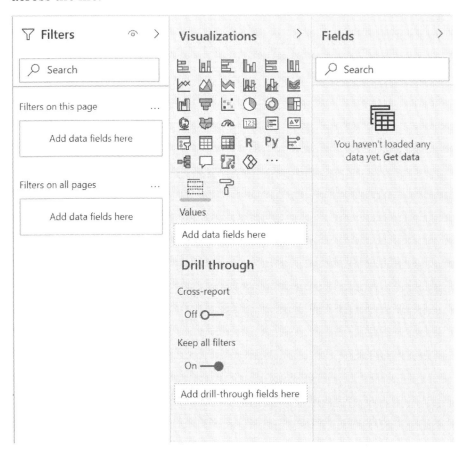

Get Started

9. Click on the arrow to hide the **Filters** pane.

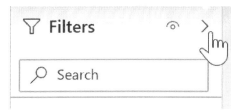

Chapter 2

Get Data

With Power BI you can connect to different data sources and types. You can use basic data sources such as CSV files and spreadsheets, or online services such as Azure, Salesforce, Dynamics, and much more.

1. Go to the File tab and save the file as Power BI Academy – Patient Dashboard.

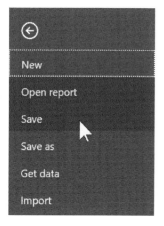

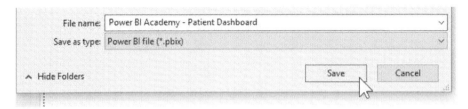

2. Visit the address **createandlearn.net/healthcare2a** and download the file **PatientData.xlsx**. This file contains the data that you will use to create the dashboard.

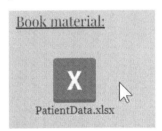

3. Go to **Home** tab and click on **Get Data**. Then, select **Excel**.

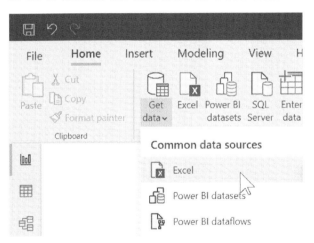

Get Data

4. Select the **PatientData.xlsx** that you have saved and click **OK**.

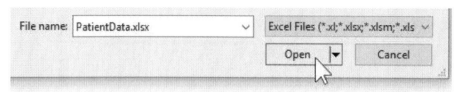

5. The Navigator window will show all available tables. Select all of them by checking their boxes and click on **Load**.

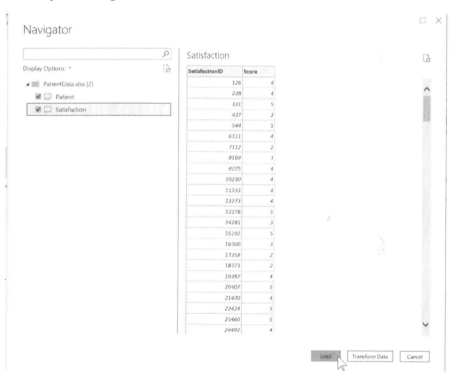

6. In the **Report** view, you will note that the **Fields** list contains every table and columns imported (Patient and Satisfaction). You can expand them by clicking on the Chevron.

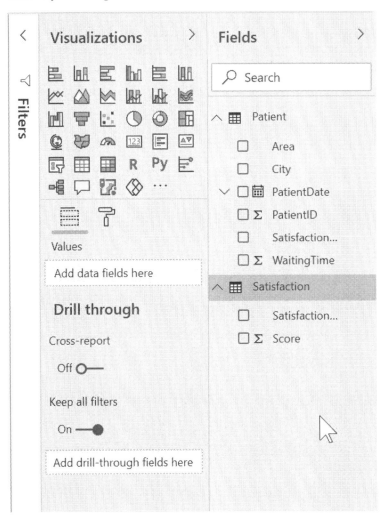

Chapter 3
Model data

With Power BI you can combine data from multiple sources and set their relationship. You can also create custom columns and calculations, making your life much easier and your reports more powerful.

1. Go to **Model** (Relationships) view.

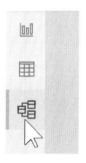

2. To define how **Patient** and **Satisfaction** will be related. Go to Home tab and click on **Manage Relationships**.

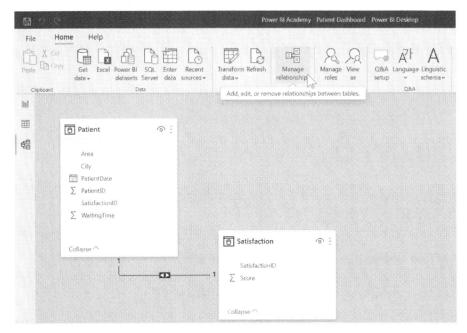

3. Power BI has already created a relationship, but we will create a new one from scratch. In the **Manage relationships** window, select the relationship created and click on **Delete**.

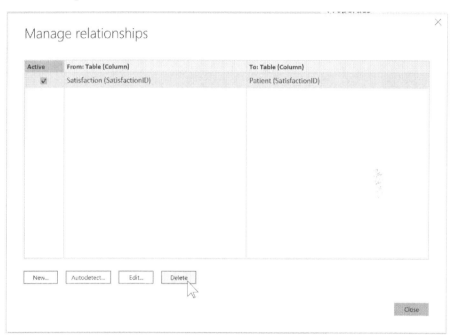

4. Click on **New**.

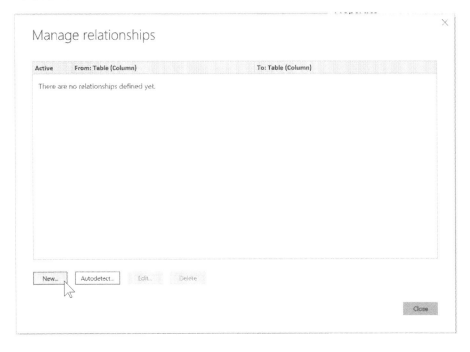

Model data

5. Select **Patient** as the top table to be related and **Satisfaction** as the second one.
To relate columns, click on them and they will be highlighted. The example below shows that SatisfactionID(Patient) will be related to SatisfactionID(Satisfaction) (BE SURE TO SELECT BOTH COLUMNS).

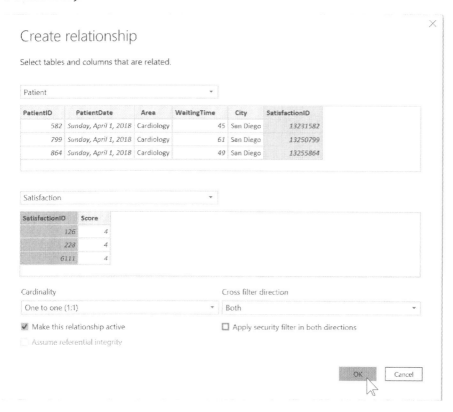

6. For cardinality, select **One to one (1:1)**, it means that every single patient record will connect to a single satisfactionID and score. Click **OK**.

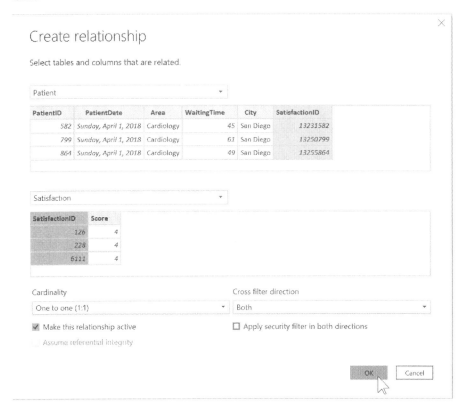

Model data

7. The relationships should look like the image below. Click on **Close**.

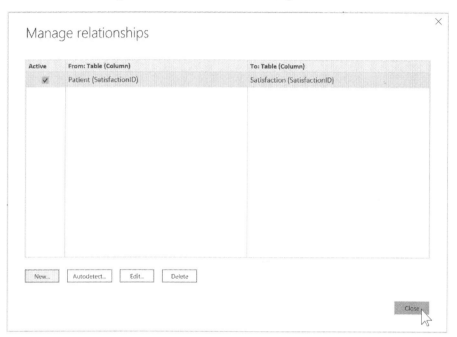

8. The relationship diagram should look like the image below. You can also move the boxes by dragging them. Click on the box title to drag each box.

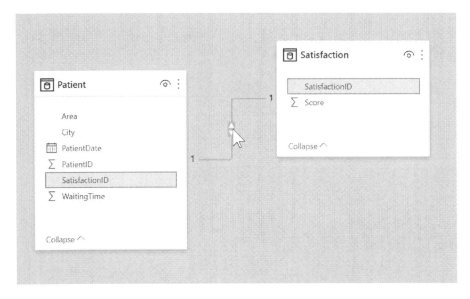

Chapter 4

Creating Custom Calculations

You can create calculated columns and measures in Power BI with Data Analysis Expressions (DAX) formulas.

DAX formulas are like Excel formulas. In fact, DAX has many of the same functions as Excel. However, DAX functions are meant to work over data interactively sliced or filtered in a report, like in Power BI Desktop.

1. Go to **Report**.

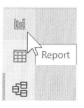

2. Go to **Fields** and select **Satisfaction**.

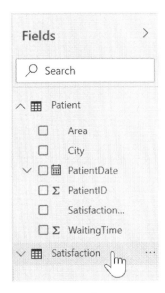

3. To create the Average of Satisfaction Score, click on **New Measure**.

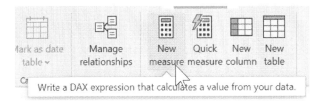

Creating Custom Calculations

4. In the formula bar, type the following formula

avg Satisfaction = sum(Satisfaction[Score])/ COUNT(Satisfaction[SatisfactionID])

Press Enter.

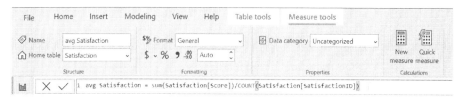

See the explanation:

avg Satisfaction = sum(Satisfaction[Score]) / COUNT(Satisfaction[SatisfactionID])
— Measure Name — Sum of **Score** field — Division — Count the numbers of **SatisfactionID**

5. The new measure is now ready to use in the **Field** list.

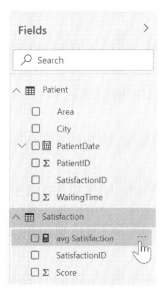

6. Go to **Fields** and select **Patient**.

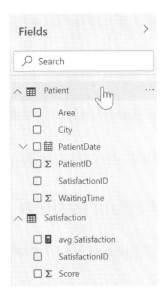

7. Right-click the **Patient** table and click on **New Measure**.

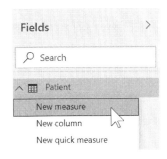

Creating Custom Calculations

8. In the formula bar, type the following formula

Patient Total = COUNTROWS(Patient)

Press Enter.

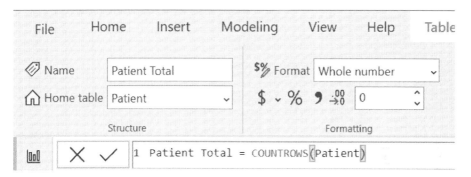

See the explanation:

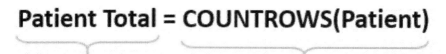

Creating Custom Calculations

Important note on FEBRUARY 2022 UPDATE:
This book was updated in 2021, and starting with the February 2022 release of Power BI Desktop, the redesigned Format pane is on by default.

This update will not impact this book's usage but is worth knowing that some icons have changed place and other visual elements have been updated.

Here are the main changes you will find:

1. Microsoft has updated the **format** tab icon and added a descriptive subtitle to make it easier to find the Format pane.

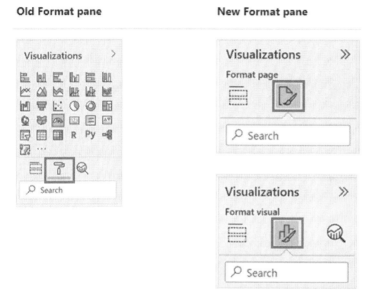

2. Microsoft moved the **Visualization** types gallery to be present only on the **Build** tab.

Old Format pane   **New Format pane**

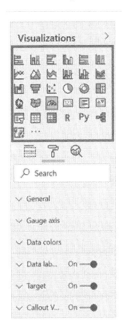 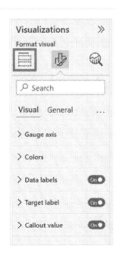

Creating Custom Calculations 41

3. Microsoft has split the long list of formatting cards into two categories: **visual** specific vs. **general** settings.

Old Format pane   **New Format pane**

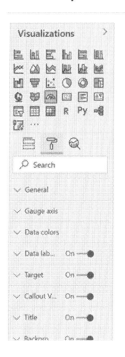
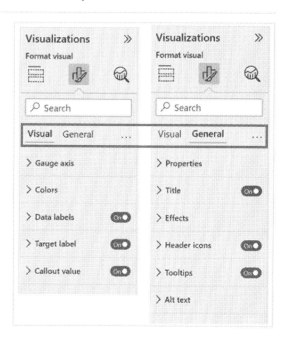

www.createandlearn.net

4. You'll notice that Microsoft has broken up the settings further into subcategories within the cards.

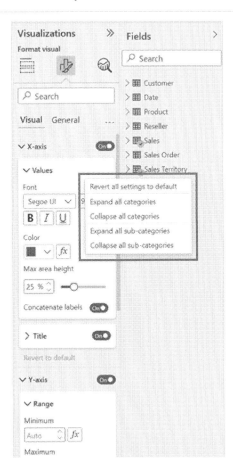

As you see, Microsoft has updated minor visual items on the formatting pane that will improve the user experience without harming any previous functionality found in this book.

Chapter 5
Dashboard Page

1. Click on a blank area on the canvas to select the page. Now you can edit the canvas.

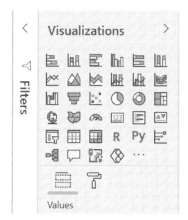

2. Go to **Visualizations**, and click on **Format**.

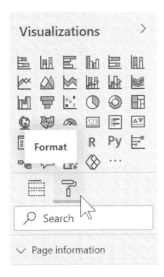

Dashboard Page

3. Go to **Page Background**, **Color,** and choose White 10% Darker), and **Transparency** of 70%.

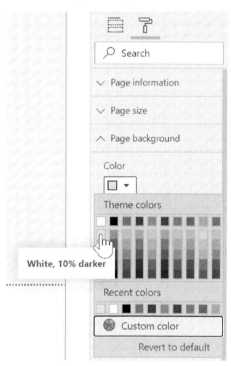

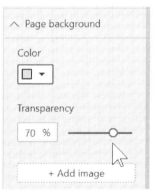

www.createandlearn.net

4. Go to Page information and change the Name field to Patient Overview.

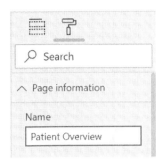

5. Go to **Page** size and set **Type** 16:9.

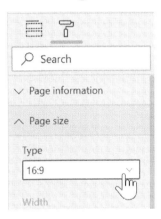

Dashboard Page

6. Visit the address **createandlearn.net/healthcare2a** and download the **five** images available. Click on the **download** icon on each image.

7. Go to Go to **Insert tab** and click on **Image**.

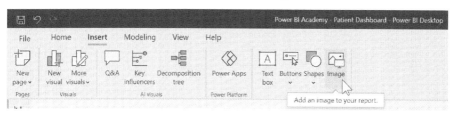

8. Select the image **HealthHeader.jpg** and click **Open**.

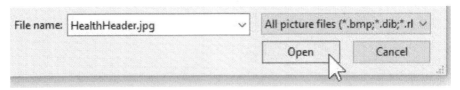

9. Go to **Format image, General,** and change the **X Position** to 0, **Y Position** to 0, **Width** to 1280, and **Height** to 201.

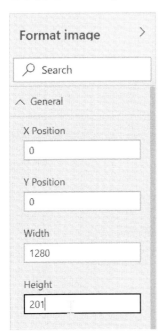

10. Go to **Scaling** and select **Fill**.

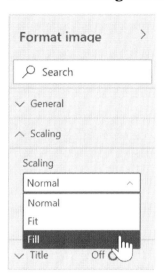

11. Go to **Format** tab and click **Send to back**.

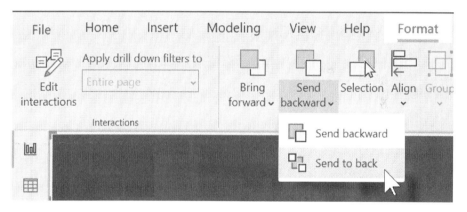

12. Go to **View** tab and click on **Themes**. Select the theme **Classroom**.

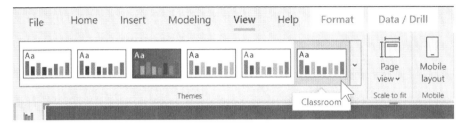

13. **Save** your file.

14. Your file should look like the image below.

Chapter 6

Big Numbers

1. Go to **Insert** tab and click on **Image**.

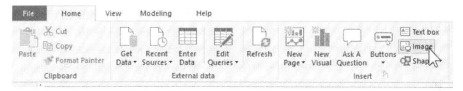

2. Select the image **Patient.png**

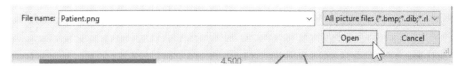

3. Go to **General** and change the **X position** to 30, **Y Position** to 120, **Width** to 50, and **Height** to 50.

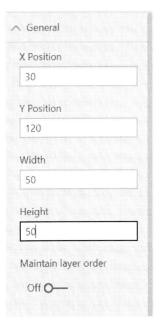

4. Go to **Insert** tab and click on **Image**.

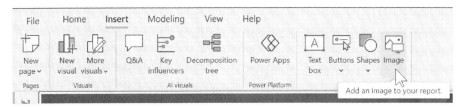

5. Select the image **Time.png**

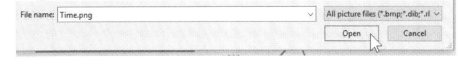

Big Numbers

6. Go to **General** and change the **X position** to 298, **Y Position** to 120, **Width** to 50, and **Height** to 50.

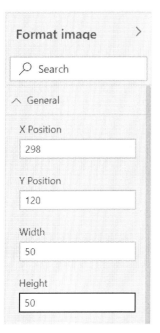

7. Go to **Insert** tab and click on **Image**.

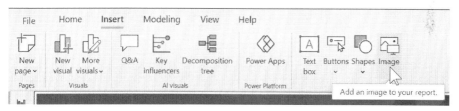

8. Select the image **Satisfaction.png**

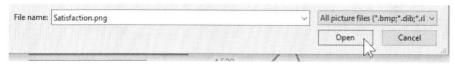

9. Go to **General** and change the **X position** to 564, **Y Position** to 120, **Width** to 50, and **Height** to 50.

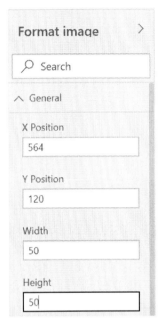

10. Click on a blank area on the canvas, to deselect the image, or just press **escape** key (Esc).

11. Go to **Visualizations** and click on **Card**.

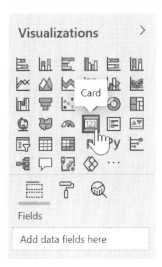

12. Power BI will create a place holder.

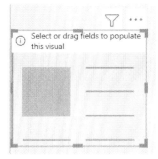

13. Drag the field PatientID from the Fields list onto the Field card component with the new card selected.

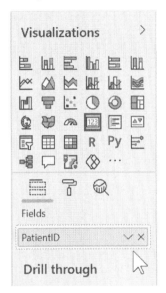

Big Numbers

14. Click on the down arrow (expand chevron) to customize the data calculation. Select **Count**. The result displayed will be the count of **PatientID**.

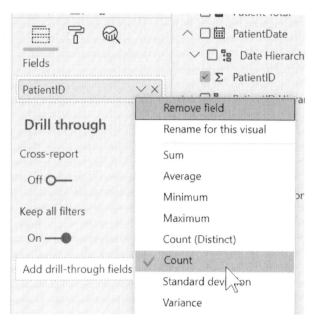

15. Click on **Format**, **Data label**, and select the color **White**.

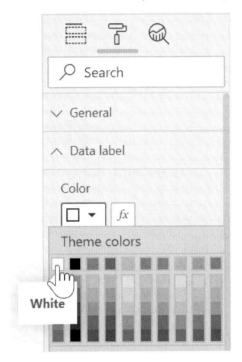

16. Change the **Text size** to 40.

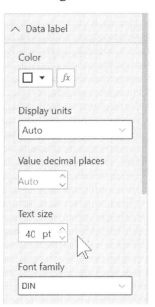

17. Switch Category label to Off, and Title to On.

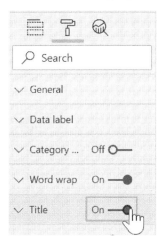

18. Go to **Title text** and type **Patients**. Change the **Font color** to white, the **Text size** to 11, and **Alignment** to Center.

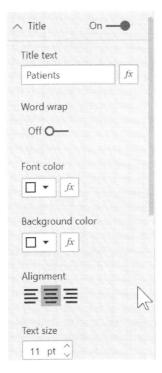

19. Go to **General** and change the **X position** to 63, **Y Position** to 90, **Width** to 190, and **Height** to 80.

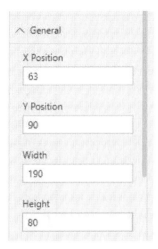

20. Note: Sometimes, you will find in the **General** group a field highlighted in red. To solve this, change all the other three fields and come back to the red one. Then, you delete and type the number again.

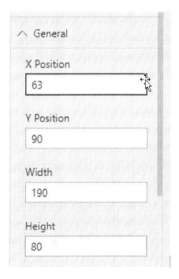

21. The new card should look like the image below.

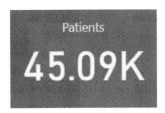

22. Select the Patients card. Then, go to **Home** tab and click on **Copy**.

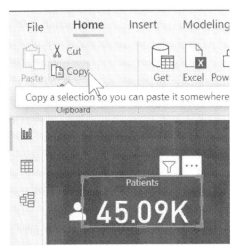

23. Click twice on **Paste** to have three identical cards.

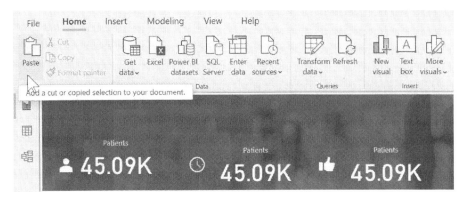

Big Numbers

24. Select the second card.

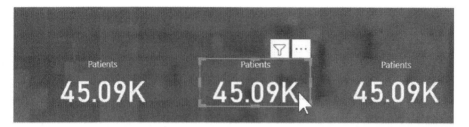

25. Change the field component to **WaitingTime**.

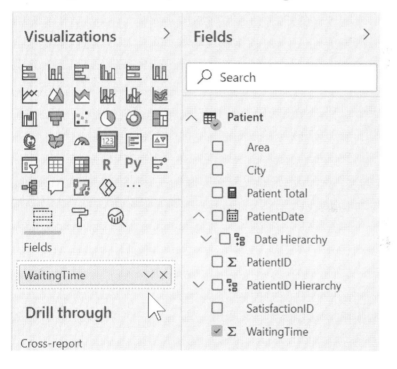

www.createandlearn.net

26. Click on the chevron and select **Average**.

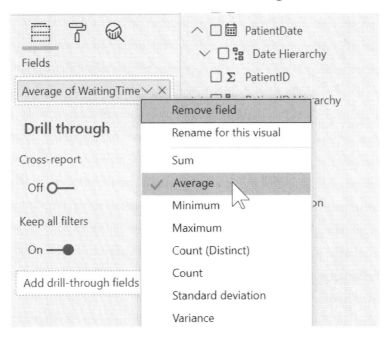

27. Go to **Format, Title,** and change the title to **Waiting Time**.

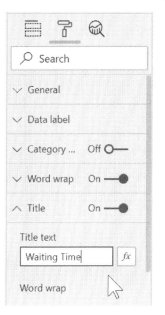

28. Go to **General** and change the **X position** to 317, **Y Position** to 90, **Width** to 190, and **Height** to 80.

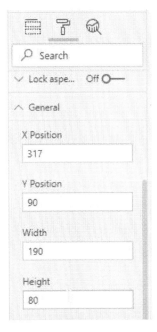

29. Select the third card.

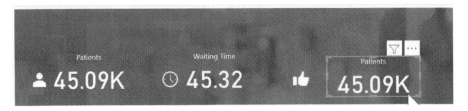

Big Numbers

30. Change the field component to **Score**.

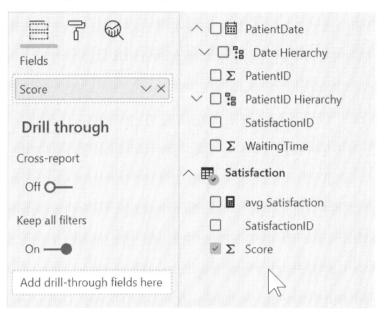

31. Click on the chevron and select **Average**.

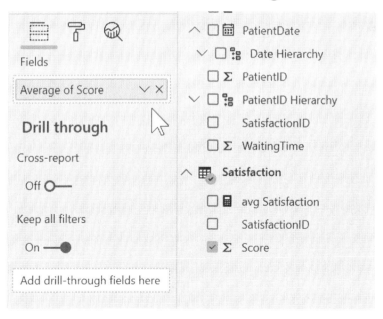

32. Go to **General** and change the **X position** to 571, **Y Position** to 90, **Width** to 190, and **Height** to 80.

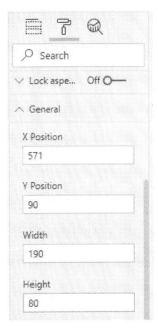

33. Go to **Format, Title,** and change the title to **Satisfaction**.

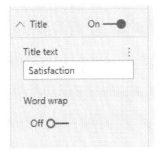

34. **Save** your file.

35. Your dashboard should look like the image below.

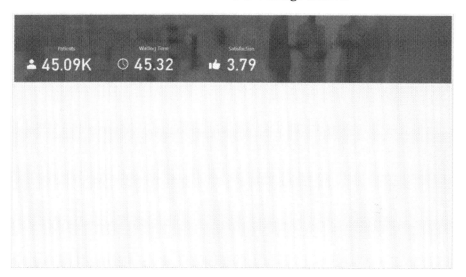

Chapter 7

Patients by Area

1. Click on a blank area on the canvas.
2. Go to Visualizations and click on Stacked bar chart.

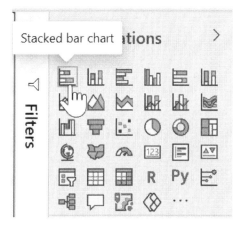

3. Drag the **Area** field to the **Axis** component. Then, drag the **PatientID** field to the **Values** component. Go to **Values**, click on the Chevron, and select **Count**.

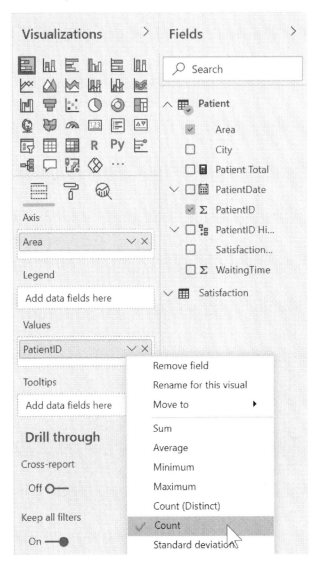

4. Go to **Format**, and switch the **X axis** to **Off**.

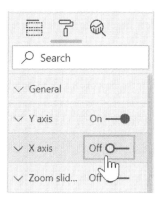

5. Switch the **Data labels** to **ON**.

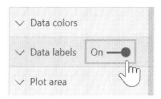

6. Go to Title, and change the Title text to **Patients by Area**. Then, change the Font color to White, 60% darker.

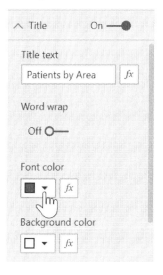

7. Go to **General** and change the **X position** to 10, **Y Position** to 200, **Width** to 300, and **Height** to 235.

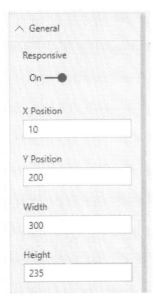

8. **Save** your file.

9. Your dashboard should look like the image below.

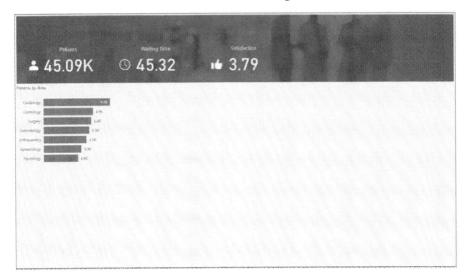

Chapter 8

Patients by Month

1. Click on a blank area on the canvas.

2. Go to Visualizations and click on Line chart.

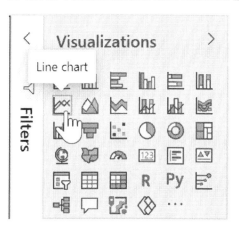

3. Drag the **Moth** of **PatientDate** field to the **Axis** component. Then, drag the **PatientID** field to the **Values** component. Go to **Values**, click on the Chevron, and select **Count**.

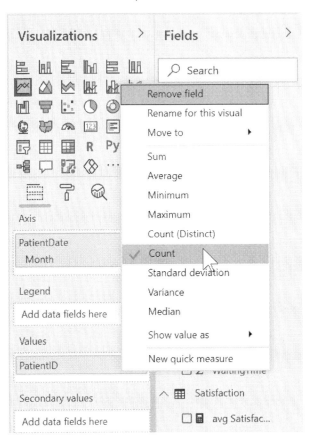

4. Go to **Format**, **Title**, and change the title to **Patients by Month**. Then, change the **Font color** to **White, 60% darker**.

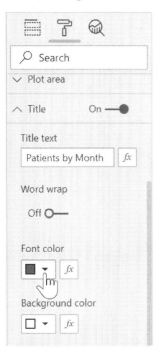

5. Go to **General** and change the **X position** to 314, **Y Position** to 200, **Width** to 550, and **Height** to 235.

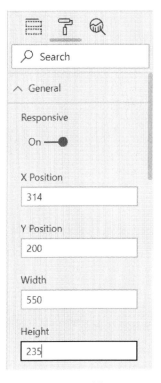

6. **Save** your file.

7. Your dashboard should look like the image below.

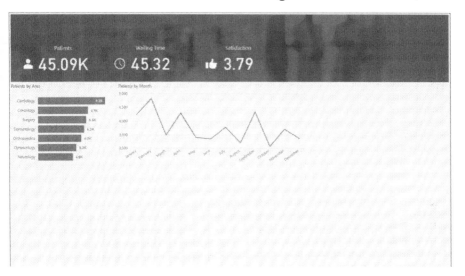

Chapter **9**

Patient Satisfaction

1. Click on a blank area on the canvas.

2. Go to Visualizations and click on Donut chart.

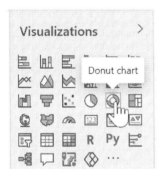

3. Drag the **Score** field to the **Legend** component. Then, drag the **Score** field to the **Values** component.

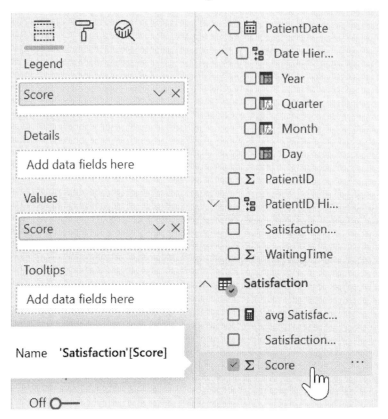

4. Go to **Format**, **Shapes**, and change the **Inner radius** to 75.

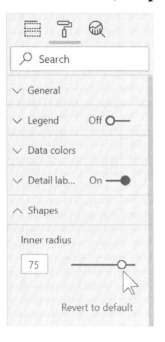

5. Switch the **Background** to **Off**. Then, go to **General** and change the **X position** to 10, **Y Position** to 450, **Width** to 300, and **Height** to 260.

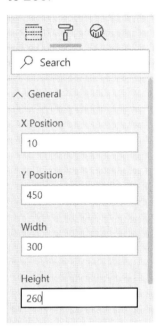

6. Go to Format, Title, and change the title to **Patient Satisfaction**. Then, change the Font color to White, 60% darker.

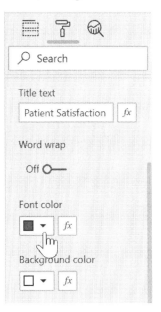

7. Click on a blank area on the canvas.

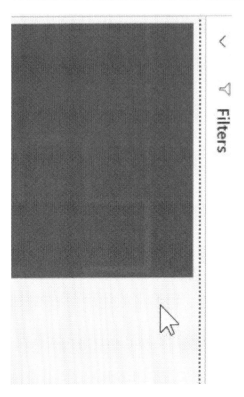

8. Go to **Visualizations** and select **Card**.

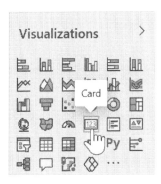

9. Drag the **avgSatisfaction** field to **Fields** component.

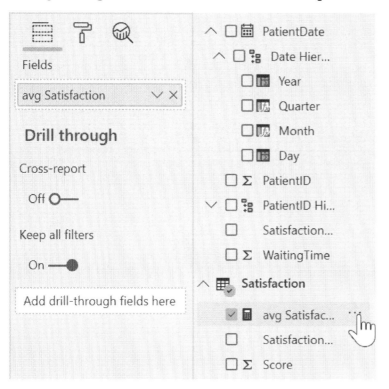

10. Go to **Format** and switch **Category label** to **Off**.

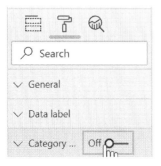

11. Go to **Data label** and change the **Text size** to 30.

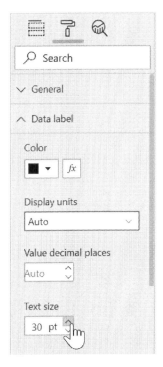

Patient Satisfaction

12. Go to **General** and change the **X position** to 91, **Y Position** to 535, **Width** to 139, and **Height** to 95.

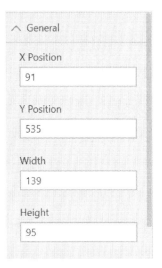

13. **Save** your file.

14. Your dashboard should look like the image below.

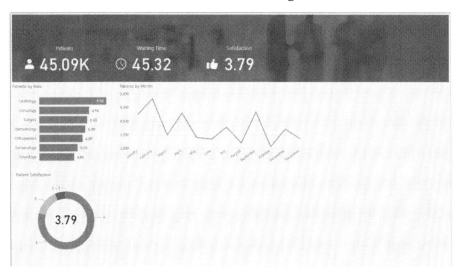

Chapter 10

Patient Table

1. Click on a blank area on the canvas.

2. Go to **Visualizations** and click on **Table**.

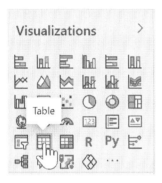

3. Drag the **Area**, **Patient Total**, **avgSatisfaction**, and **Waiting time** field to the **Values** component.

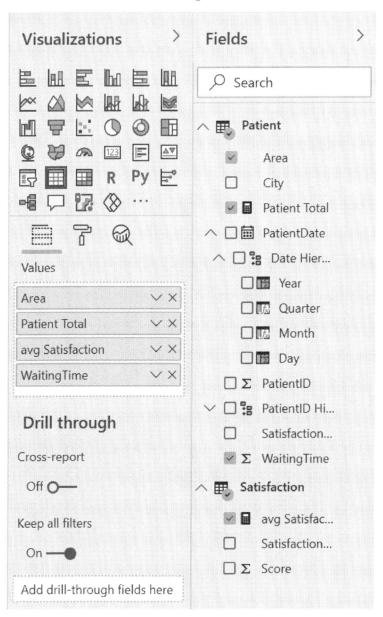

4. Go to **Waiting Time** and change the calculation to **Average**.

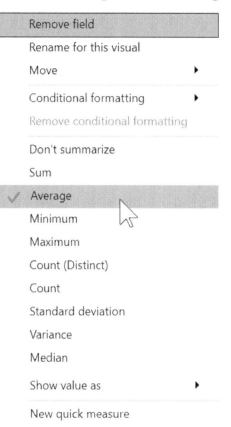

5. Go to **General** and change the **X position** to 314, **Y Position** to 450, **Width** to 550, and **Height** to 260.

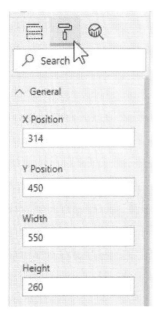

6. Go to **Format**, **Style,** and change to **None**.

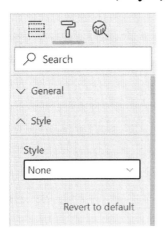

7. Switch the **Vertical grid** and the **Horizontal grid** to **Off**. Then, change **Row padding** to 4.

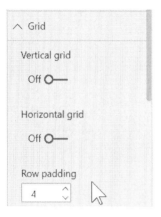

8. Go to **Column headers** and change the **Text size** to 10.

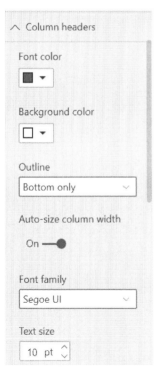

9. Go to **Values** and change the **Text size** to 10.

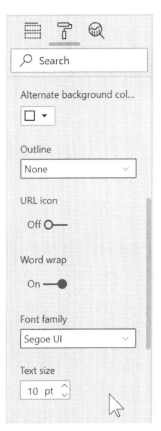

10. Go to **Conditional formatting** and select **Average of WaitingTime.**

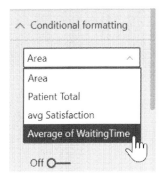

11. Switch **Data bars** to **On**.

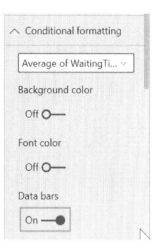

12. Click on Advanced controls.

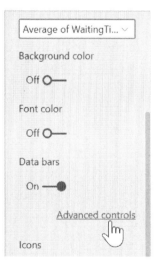

13. The **Data bars** window will appear. Change the **Positive bar** and **Negative bar** color to #b7d1f1 (light blue). Then, click **OK**.

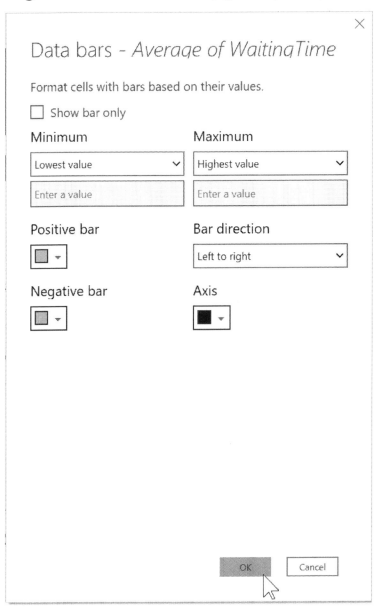

14. Go to **Fields**, **avgSatisfaction** and click on the **More options** (ellipsis).

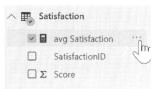

15. Click on **Rename** and change the name to **Average of Satisfaction**.

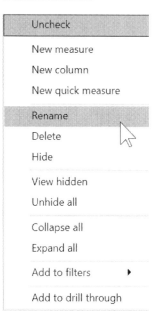

16. Click on **Average of Waiting Time** column title to change the sort option.

Area	Patient Total	Average of Satisfaction	Average of Waiting Time
Cardiology	9261	4.09	5.17
Gynaecology	5257	3.78	45.41
Surgery	6616	3.76	46.44
Dermatology	6337	3.76	46.87
Concology	6866	3.76	47.90
Neurology	4792	3.75	49.97
Orthopaedics	5958	3.45	51.41
Total	45087	3.79	45.32

17. **Save** your file.

18. Your dashboard should look like the image below.

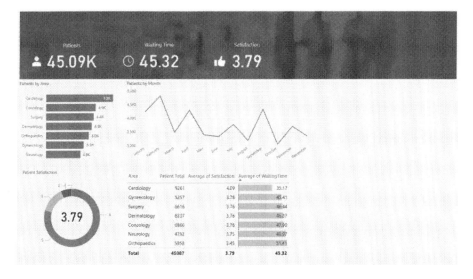

Chapter **11**

Patient by City

1. Click on a blank area on the canvas.

2. Go to **Visualizations** and click on **Map**.

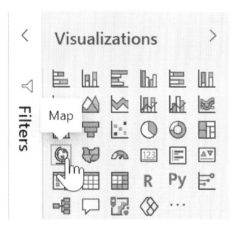

3. Drag the **City** field to the **Location** component. Then, drag the **PatientID** field to the **Size** component. Go to **PatientID**, click on the Chevron, and select **Count**.

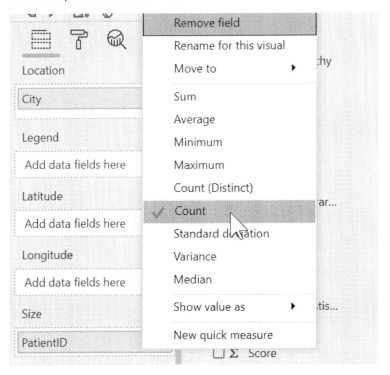

4. Go to **Format**, **Bubbles,** and change the **Size** to 30.

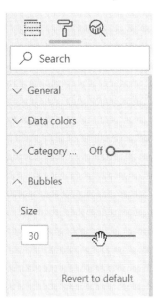

5. Go to **Map styles** and select **Light**.

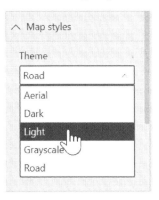

6. Go to **Format**, **Title**, and change the title to **Total Patient by City**. Then, change the Font color to White, 60% darker.

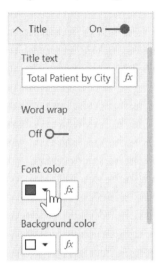

7. Go to **General** and change the **X position** to 872, **Y Position** to 450, **Width** to 400, and **Height** to 260.

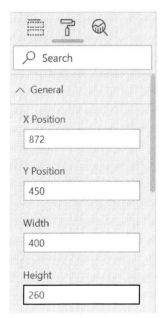

8. **Save** your file.
9. Your dashboard should look like the image below.

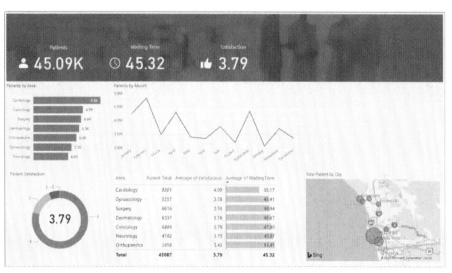

Chapter 12
Waiting Time

1. Click on a blank area on the canvas.

2. Go to **Visualizations** and click on **Get More Visuals** (ellipsis).

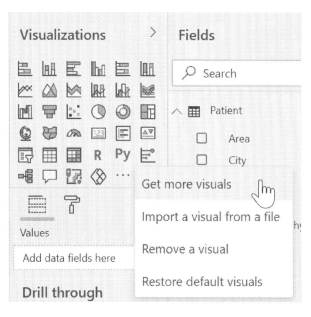

3. Select Get More Visuals

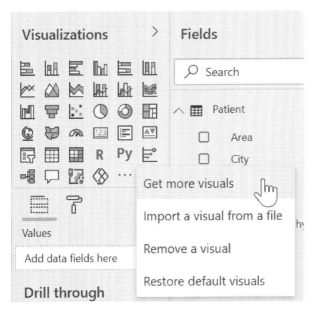

4. Sign in with your Power BI account or select **Try for free**.

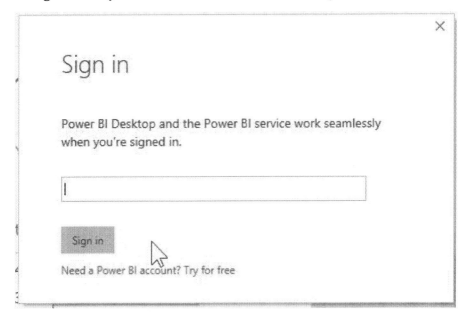

5. The marketplace has a big list of free visuals, and it is continuously updated. Search for **Radar**.

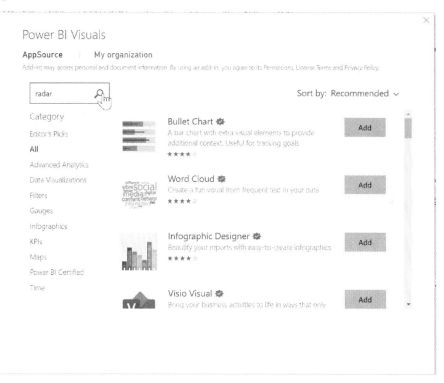

6. When you find the **Radar Chart** click on **Add**.

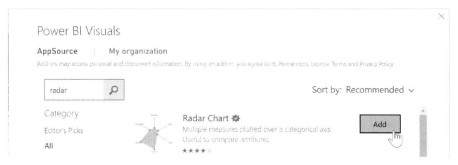

7. Click **OK**.

Import custom visual

The visual was successfully imported into this report.

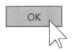

8. Now I have a new item on my **Visualizations** pane called **Radar Chart 1.3.1**. Click on **Radar**.

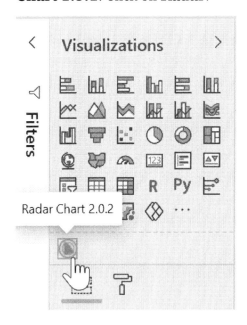

9. Drag the **Area** field to the **Category** component. Then, drag the **WaitingTime** field to the **Y Axis** component.

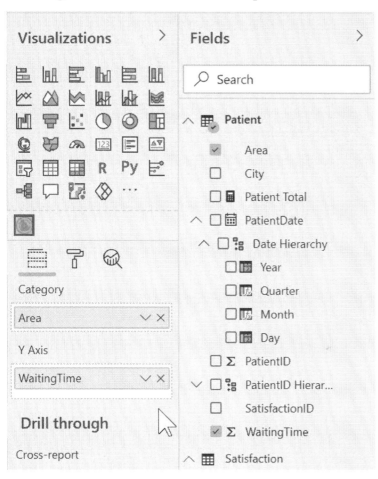

10. Go to **WaitingTime**, click on the Chevron, and select **Average**.

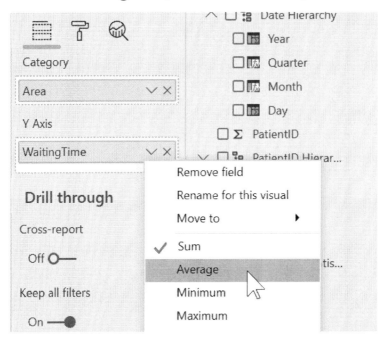

11. Go to **Format**, **Title**, and change the title to **Waiting Time by Area**. Then, change the Font color to White, 60% darker.

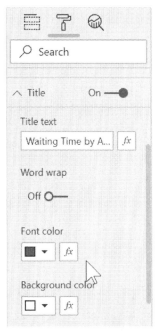

12. Go to **Legend** and switch to **Off**.

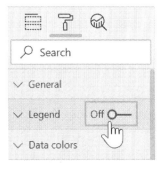

13. Go to **General** and change the **X position** to 872, **Y Position** to 201, **Width** to 400, and **Height** to 235.

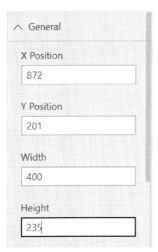

14. Your dashboard should look like the image below.

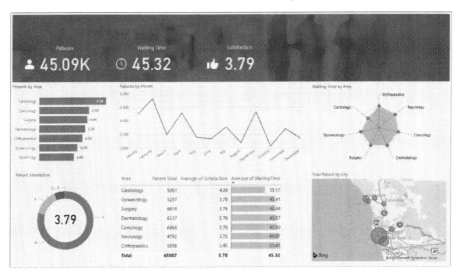

Chapter 13

Filters

1. Click on a blank area on the canvas.

2. Go to **View** tab, **Show panes,** and click on **Selection.**

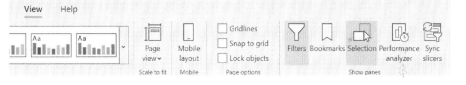

3. On **Selection,** the **Image** (header) object needs to be at the bottom.

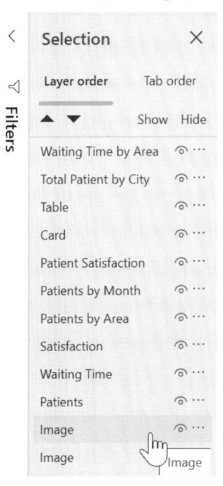

Filters

4. You can use the arrows to move the **Layer order** if needed.

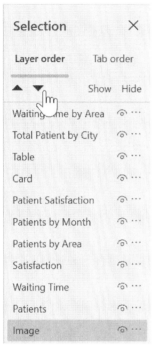

5. Go to **View** tab and uncheck the **Selection** pane.

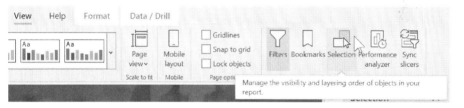

6. Go to Visualizations and click on Slicer.

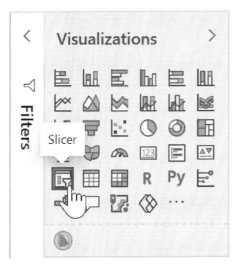

7. Drag the **PatientDate** field to the **Field** component.

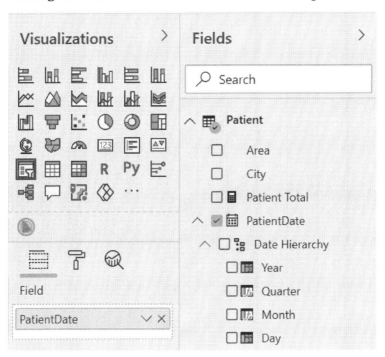

Filters

8. Go to **General** and change the **X position** to 772, **Y Position** to 83, **Width** to 300, and **Height** to 106.

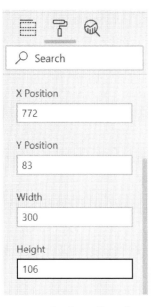

9. Switch the **Slice header** to **Off**.

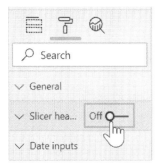

10. Go to **Date inputs** and change the **Font color** to **White**.

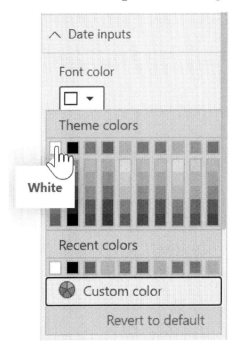

11. Go to **Slider** and change the **Color** to White, 10% darker.

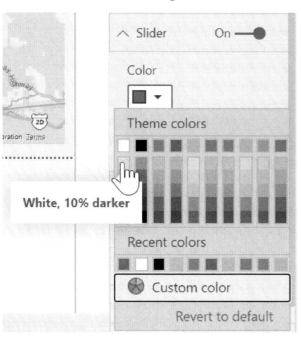

12. Swicth the **Title** to On, and change the **Title text** to **Date**. Then, change the **Font color** to **White**.

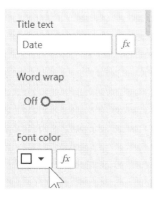

13. Click on a blank area on the canvas.

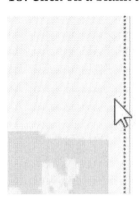

14. Go to **Visualizations** and click on **Slicer**.

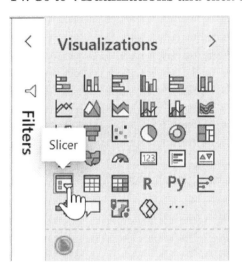

Filters

15. Drag the **City** field to the **Field** component.

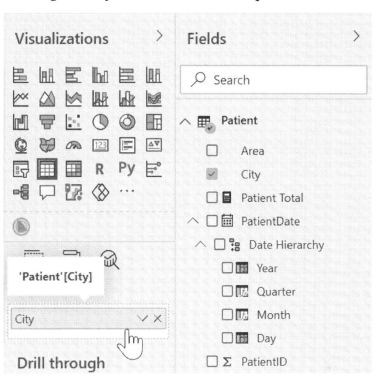

16. Go to **General** and change the **X position** to 1090, **Y Position** to 66, **Width** to 166, and **Height** to 125.

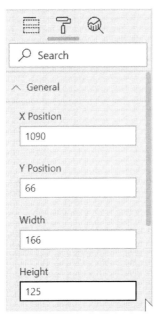

17. Switch the **Title** to On and **Slicer head** to off.

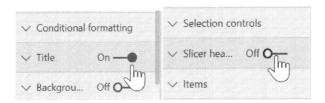

18. Change the **Title text** to **City** and the **Font color** to **white**.

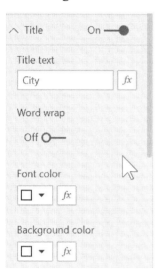

19. Go to **Items**, **Font color,** and change to **White**.

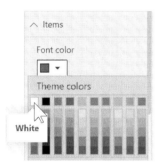

20. **Save** your file.

21. Your dashboard should look like the image below.

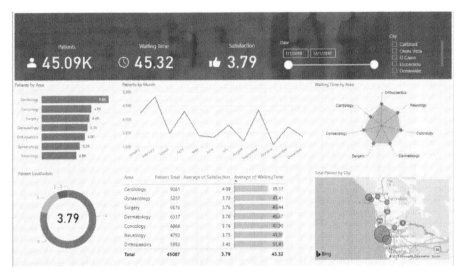

Chapter 14

Text and Objects

1. Click on a blank area on the canvas.

2. Go to **Insert** tab and click on **Text box**.

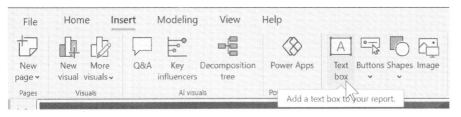

3. In the new text box, type **Patient Overview Dashboard**.

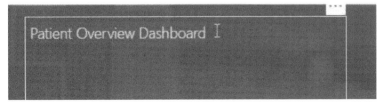

4. Select the text and change the **text size** to 20, **Bold**, and **text color** white.

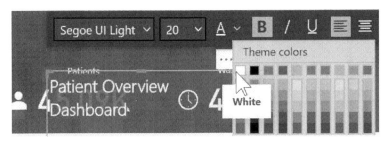

5. Go to **General** and change the **X position** to 16, **Y Position** to 28, **Width** to 358, and **Height** to 55.

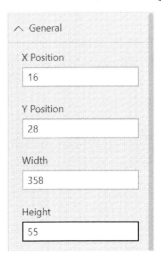

Text and Objects   129

6. Go to **Insert** tab, **Shapes,** and click on **Line**.

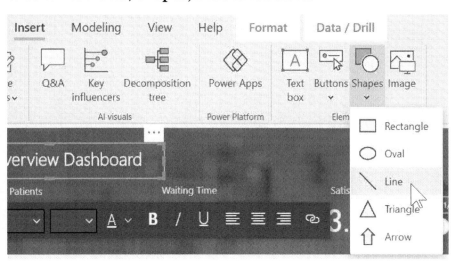

7. Go to **Format shape**, **Rotation,** and change to 90 degrees.

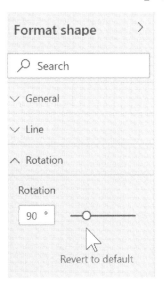

www.createandlearn.net

8. Go to **General** and change the **X position** to 8, **Y Position** to 45, **Width** to 720, and **Height** to 56.

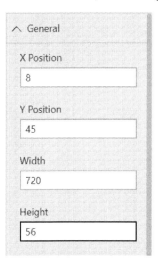

9. Go to **Line**, and change the **Line color** to **white**. Then, change the **Weight** to 2.

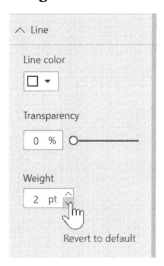

10. **Save** your file.

11. **Congratulations**! Your Dashboard is finished and ready to be shared or published.

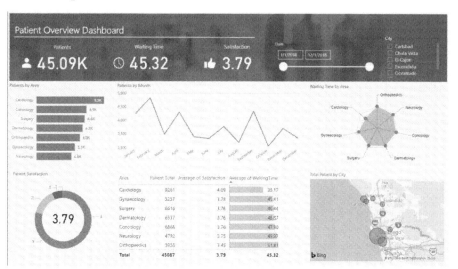

Chapter 15

Bookmarks

In Power BI you can use bookmarks to capture a specific configured view, including visuals and filters.

It is useful to create a **Clean Filter** effect or to create a collection of bookmarks to be presented in a story sequence.

1. Go to **View** tab and select **Bookmarks Pane**.

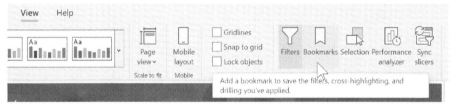

2. Go to the **Bookmarks** pane and click on **Add**.

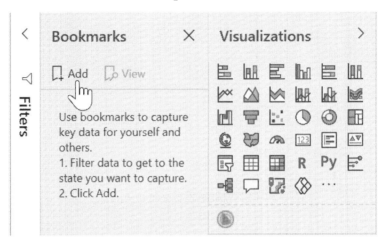

3. Double-click the **Bookmark 1** and type the new name **MainBookmark**.

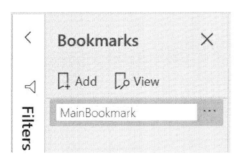

4. Close the Bookmarks pane.

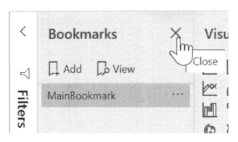

5. Go to **Insert** tab, and click on **Image**.

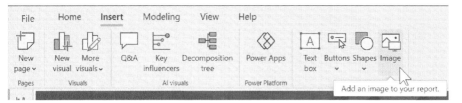

6. Select the image **Filter.png** and click on **Open**.

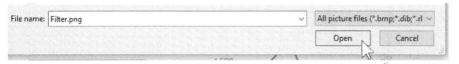

7. Go to **General** and change the **X position** to 1224, **Y Position** to 8, **Width** to 48, and **Height** to 40.

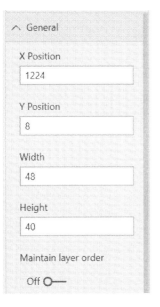

8. Switch **Action** to **On**.

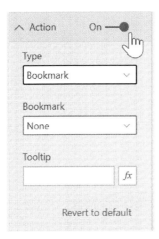

9. Go to **Type** and select **Bookmark**. Then, go to **Bookmark** and select **MainBookmark**.

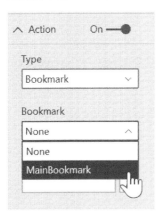

10. Your dashboard should look like the image below.

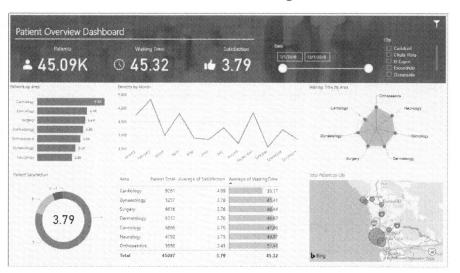

11. Go to **Date** filter and change the end date to June 30th.

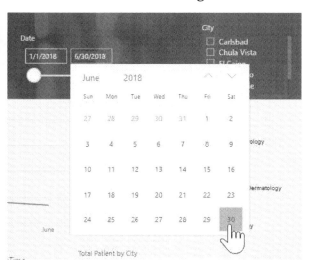

12. Go to **City** filter, and change to **San Diego**.

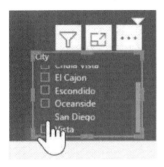

13. Go to **Patient Satisfaction** and click on score 5.

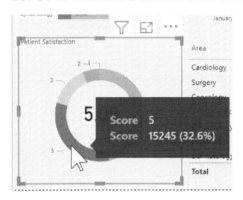

14. Now the dashboard is using multiple filters and slicers.

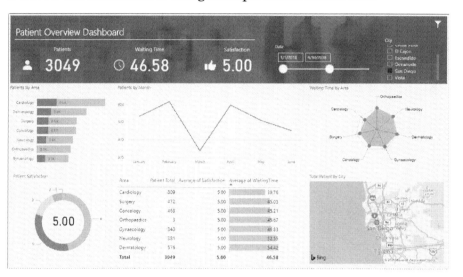

15. To return to the first bookmark created, hold **CTRL** key and **click** on the **filter** image.

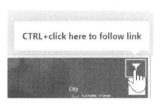

16. The dashboard filters and slicers have returned to the previous configuration.

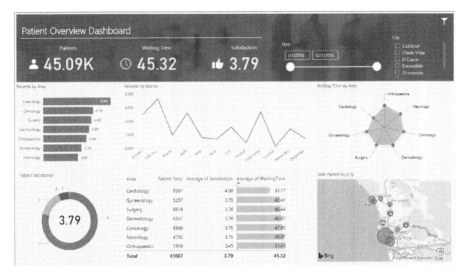

17. **Save** your file.

18. Your dashboard should look like the image below.

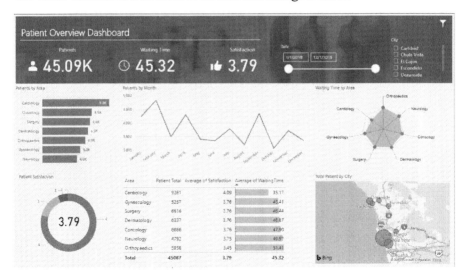

Chapter 16

Phone Layout

1. To create a mobile dashboard, go to **View** tab, and click on **Mobile Layout**.

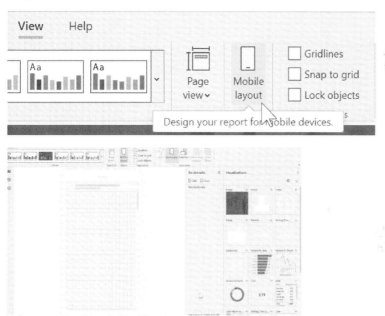

2. Move the **visual** from **Visualizations** pane into the mobile layout. You can resize and change the order the way you want.

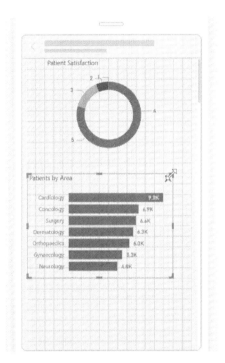

3. To go back, click on **Mobile Layout** (Switch to Desktop Layout).

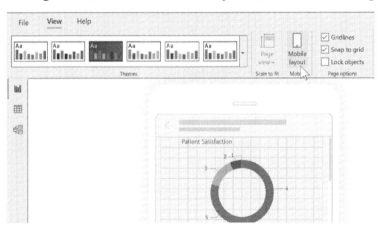

4. **Save** your file.

Chapter 17

Sharing

1. To export your Dashboard to PDF, go to the **File** tab and click on **Export to PDF**.

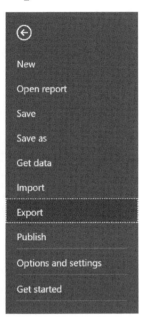
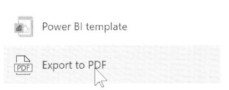

2. Power BI will create a PDF file that you can save and share.

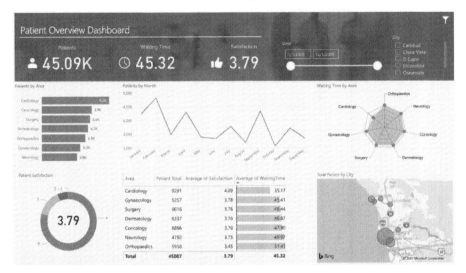

3. To publish in Power BI service go to **File** tab and click on **Publish**.

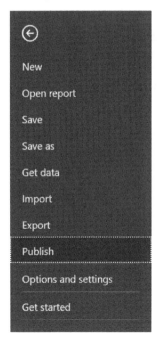

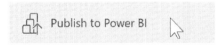

4. Power BI will ask if you want to save any changes before publishing. Click on **Save**.

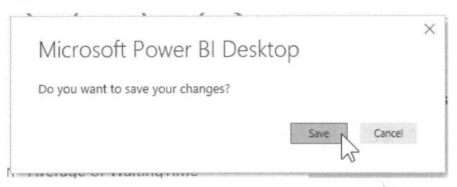

5. Select the destination (My workspace) and click on **Select**.

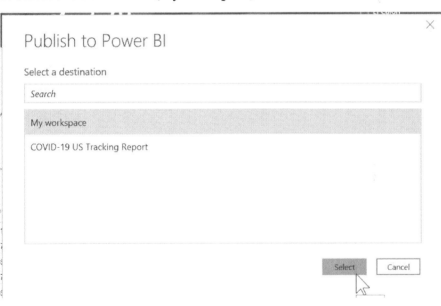

6. Power BI will publish your Dashboard.

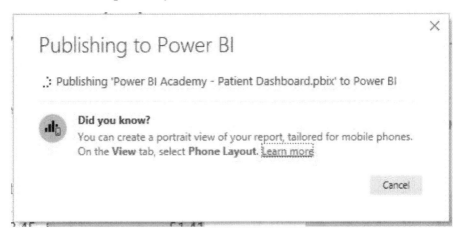

7. When it is done, click on Open' Power BI academy – Patient Dashboard.pbix' in Power BI.

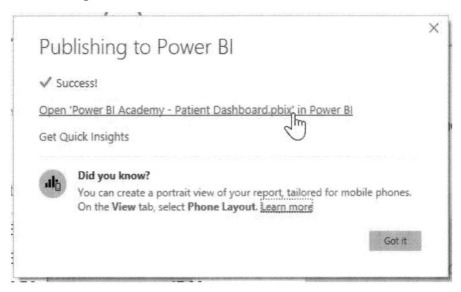

8. Sign In with your account if you need to.

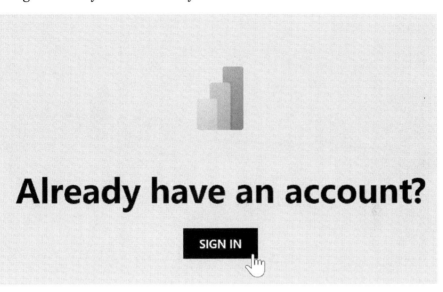

9. The Dashboard created in Power BI Desktop will sit in the **My workspace** and in the **Reports** area. Select it.

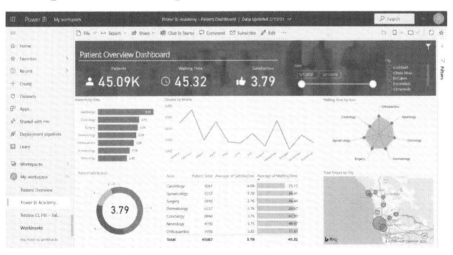

10. In Power BI service you will find more options to export your reports such as **PowerPoint**, **PDF,** and **Print**. Go to Export, and click on **PowerPoint**.

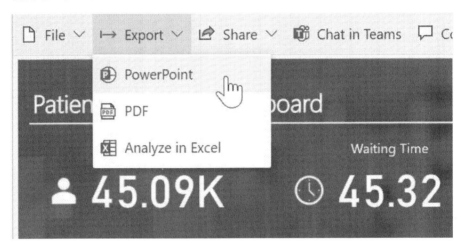

11. Select Export with Current Values and click on Export.

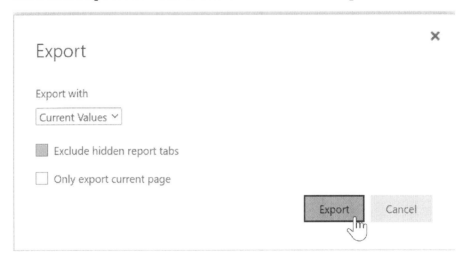

12. Power BI will create a PowerPoint file with a slide cover and all the visuals.

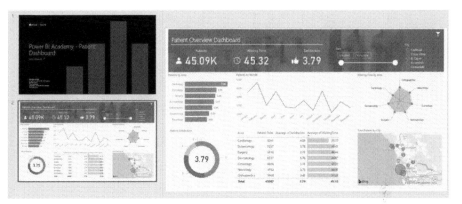

13. If you have a Power BI Pro account, you can use the **Share** button to share your work with others in your organization.

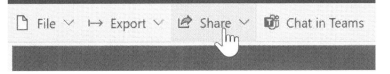

14. Here you have the option to insert the email from a company member and share your Dashboard. Note that you can customize a message of invitation, and limit if the user can share your material.

Share report
POWER BI ACADEMY – PATIENT DASHBOARD

Share   Access

Recipients will have the same access as you unless row-level security on the dataset further restricts them. Learn more

Grant access to

Enter email addresses

Include an optional message...

☑ Allow recipients to share your report
☑ Allow recipients to build new content using the underlying datasets
☑ Send an email notification to recipients

Report link ⓘ

https://app.powerbi.com/groups/me/reports/a71ad7be-a6b8-433f-afa6-d3a73c6

Share   Cancel

15. To Publish your dashboard to the web click on the **share**, **Embed report** and select **Publish to web (public)**. Note that this option generates a link that anyone can access, this should **not** be used if you have sensitive information that should not be shared to the public.

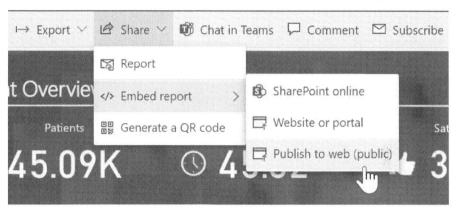

16. Power BI will show an alert about publishing on a public website. To create an embed code, click on **Create embed code**.

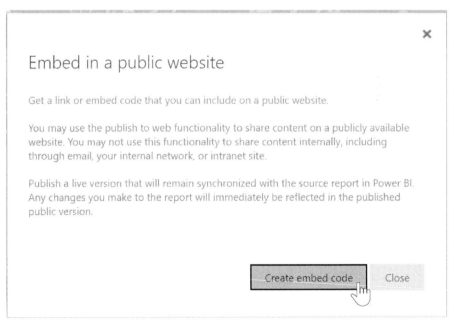

17. Click on **Publish** to create the code.

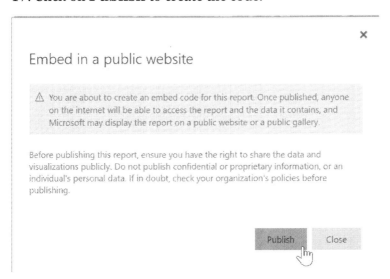

18. It will generate an embed code that you can include in your website. *Note that this will share to the public, it is not recommended to use this function when you have sensitive data.

19. You can share through a link or use an html code. Also, you can select the size.

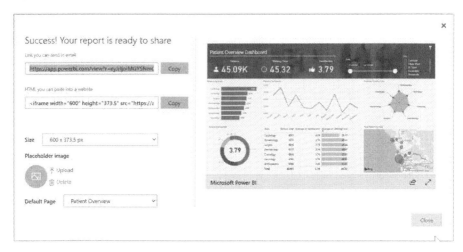

Next Steps

This book was created to help you learn by doing and through practice and expanding your knowledge in Power BI.

If you want to practice and learn more about working with Power BI Desktop, I recommend you try the book **Power BI – Business Intelligence Clinic**.

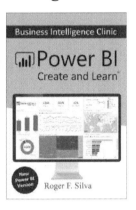

If you want to keep practicing and improving your knowledge in Power BI through several industries, I recommend the series **Power BI Academy**, where each book will introduce you to different industry metrics and datasets.

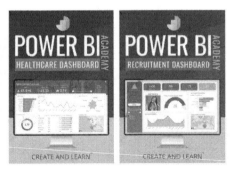

Visit the page www.createandlearn.net to have access to those books and more.

www.createandlearn.net

Final words

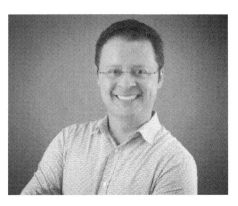

Thank you for the journey! I truly hope that you have enjoyed learning from this book as much as I have enjoyed writing and teaching the contents of this book.

Although the Business Intelligence concept is not new, the tools and methods have changed dramatically in recent years, and you made the right decision to gain more knowledge about this software.

What do you think of this book? I would like to ask you to take a minute to **review** my book. Reviews are incredibly important for my work.

If you have any comments or suggestions, please send me an email or a message and **connect with me on LinkedIn** — — I would love to hear from you and have you in my network.

Thank you for the time we spent creating and learning.

Roger F. Silva

contact.createandlearn@gmail.com
createandlearn.net
www.linkedin.com/in/roger-f-silva
You can find more Create and Learn books, files, articles, and videos:

www.createandlearn.net

https://www.createandlearn.net/

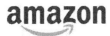

https://www.amazon.com/Roger-F-Silva/e/B07JC8J1L5/

http://www.facebook.com/createandlearn.net

https://www.linkedin.com/company/create-and-learn

https://www.instagram.com/createandlearn_net/

https://www.youtube.com/channel/UCE4BQDcEuUE9lmCZfviSZLg/featured

Final words

More **Create and Learn** books https://www.createandlearn.net/:

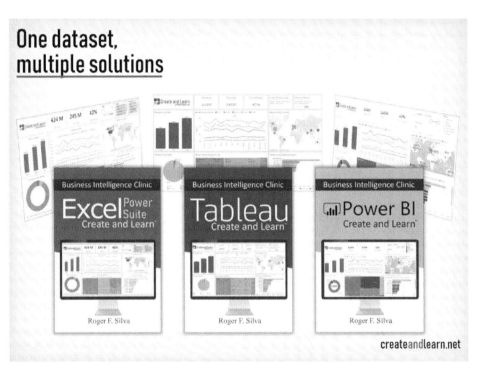

Printed by Amazon Italia Logistica S.r.l.
Torrazza Piemonte (TO), Italy